50

Frequently Asked Questions about Asbestos & Cancer

Table of Contents

Part 2

What are the effects of getting exposed to Asbestos dust?

Is it possible to be infected by asbestosis symptoms?

Do small amounts of asbestos dust cause cancer?

Is smoking related to Mesothelioma?

What are the sources of Asbestos exposure?

What are the symptoms of Asbestosis and Mesothelioma?

What diseases are caused by asbestos exposure?

Part 3

What is Multicystic Mesothelioma?

Will prolonged exposure to asbestos dust cause death?

What risks are associated with asbestos exposure?

What is Asbestos exposure?

Is asbestos exposure deadly?

How is exposure to asbestos dust treated?

What is the relationship between asbestos and lung cancer?

Part 4

How does asbestos affect health?

How fast can asbestos dust affect someone?

How long does it take for one to get Asbestos poisoning?

What are the symptoms of asbestos cancer?

How can you tell if your home is in danger of asbestos exposure?

How do you know when asbestos is in the lungs?

What are the symptoms of Asbestos in the lungs?

What are the symptoms of Asbestos inhalation?

What are the symptoms of asbestos-related diseases?

What are the symptoms of Asbestosis?

When was asbestos banned?

Does asbestos cancer have a cure?

Part 5

References

INTRODUCTION

Asbestos is a group of naturally occurring fibrous minerals that have commercial benefits due to their unusual resistance to tensile strength, poor heat conduction, and relative resistance to chemical attacks.

They were discovered long ago and widely used by the Chinese and ancient Egyptians. The word asbestos is derived from a Greek word that means combustible and degradable. In the mid-19th century, Italians were able to find ways of spinning and weaving asbestos fibers and to obtain materials that could be used in a variety of fields.

As time went on, the industry developed globally and the first laboratory for the manufacture of materials was opened in 1870 in Germany, and in 1900, asbestos found application in the manufacture of cement sheets. Today, they are used for indoor insulation and in a variety of product components, such as roofing sheets, water supply pipes, fire extinguisher blankets, plastic fillers, and medical packaging, as well as for car clutches, car brake linings, gaskets, and platforms.

The main forms of Asbestos are Chrysotile (white asbestos) and Crocidolite (blue asbestos). Other forms include Amosite, Anthophyllite, Tremolite, and Actinolite.

- **Chrysotile asbestos:** This type is obtained from serpentine rocks and is one of the most widely used in the industry. There are indications that this form of asbestos is harmful to health.
- **Brown asbestos:** Also known as Amosite Asbestos, it is known commercially as lymphocytes and is obtained from the mines of North Africa.
- **Blue Asbestos:** Rebecate is called Amphipole from Africa and Australia and it is the fibrous composition of Ampholebic Rebecate.

Over 100 million individuals worldwide are currently exposed to asbestos in their workplaces. Research has proven that all forms of asbestos are carcinogens for humans and may cause mesothelioma, lung cancer, larynx, and ovarian cancer. Exposure to this substance also leads to other diseases, such as asbestos (cirrhosis of the lungs), a plaque of the lung membranes, thickening, and effusion.

According to the estimates given by WHO, more than 107,000 people die each year from lung cancer, mesothelioma, and asbestos from workplace exposure. It is also estimated that asbestos accounts for a third of all cancer-related deaths from carcinogenicity in the workplace. It is estimated that several thousand deaths a year can be attributed to asbestos exposure at home.

The World Health Assembly resolution on cancer prevention urges the Member States to pay particular attention to the types of cancer in which avoidable exposure is a factor, including exposure to chemicals in the workplace.
In its resolution 60-26, the World Health Assembly requested the World Health Organization to undertake a global campaign to eliminate asbestos-related diseases…withstanding not to ignore a different approach to the regulation of its various forms in line with relevant international legal instruments and the most recent evidence. With effective interventions.

You will learn more about asbestos cancer in this book as 50 different frequently asked questions relating to asbestos and asbestos cancer are answered.

PART 1

1. What is Amosite Asbestos Exposure?

Amosite Asbestos is one in all six varieties of Asbestos classified on the basis of their constituent minerals in their natural states. They are fibrous in nature. Amosite is the grunerite mineral. As per the American Cancer Society, it is the most dangerous and common kind of asbestos, exposure to which can cause cancers like Lung cancer, mesothelioma and other diseases like asbestosis.

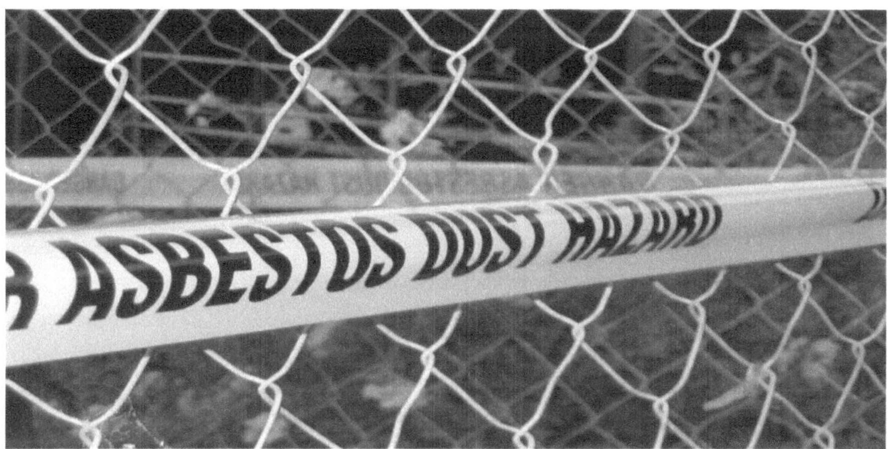

According to the National Institute for Occupational Health and Safety, around 30 % are mesothelioma cancer cases caused by exposure to amosite asbestos. As amosite is mainly used for manufacturing commercial products like cement, plumbing insulations, electrical insulations, schools, etc, the people who are majorly exposed to this are plumbers, electricians, buildings constructors, etc.

With prolonged exposure and high-intensity exposure to amosite asbestos, the chances of developing cancer are higher as with every exposure the body's autoimmune system gets affected with every cell mutation taking place inside.

2. Can Asbestos Exposure Cause Cancer?

Yes, exposure to asbestos fibers can cause a type of cancer called Mesothelioma. This disease affects a particular kind of tissue called Mesothelium. The organs of the body are covered by this thin tissue layer. Asbestos fibers when breathed in, start dwelling in this tissue and after their stay for a number of years, they start causing inflammation, injury, and malformations. This process eventually leads to cancer.

Mesothelioma cancer is categorized on the basis of the body parts it affects. Its symptoms are loss of body weight, lumps or pain in the affected area, pain while coughing and inability to breathe. Theoretically, one asbestos fiber can lead to the evolution of a single cell from which cancer can develop. Each additional exposure can, therefore, add to the cell evolution, and with each such exposure, the body's immunity is lowered. Accordingly, the more the number of times the exposure takes place, the more are the chances of developing cancer.

3.   What are Asbestos Exposure Levels?

The Occupational Safety and Health Commission (OSHA) has specified an asbestos exposure limit of the permitted level of 0.1 fiber per cubic cm. This applies to all industries like shipping, construction, etc. However, no level of exposure to asbestos is safe enough.

Mostly, people are exposed to the low levels of asbestos which is present in the air, water, and soil. So this level doesn't affect the health of people severely that can cause deadly diseases. But yet the prolonged exposure of the same can be risky.

People who are exposed to high levels of asbestos regularly do fall sick. These are those whose occupation involves the same as shipbuilding traders, asbestos miners, and millers, manufacturers of asbestos products, insulation workers, firefighters, auto parts workers, rescue and demolition workers, etc.

This is because these occupants are exposed to more asbestos released in the air for a longer period of time as well as high intensity of the exposure. Hence, the more the exposure level, the worse is the related health hazards.

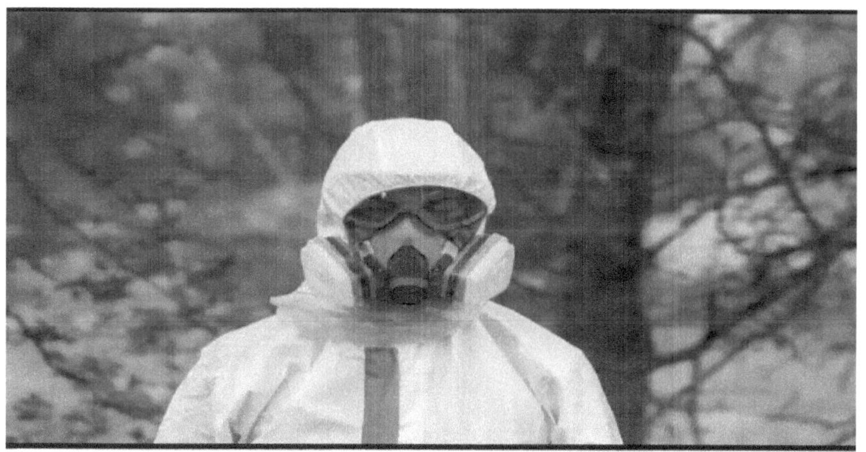

4. Can Asbestos Exposure Treatment Be Effective?

Though asbestos exposure is a permanent condition and can be fatal, however, advanced levels of treatments and therapies can eradicate its symptoms, slow down its advancement and may lead to the survival of the person for many years after the exposure and its respective diagnosis.

Treatment effectiveness depends on case to case on the basis of their diagnosis, stage, type of cancer and the current health condition and immunity of the patient to go through the treatment.

Accordingly, the kinds of treatments that can be used are medication, breathing equipment, therapies, surgeries like resection, lobectomy and Pneumonectomy, chemotherapy, radiation therapy or a combination of all known as multimodal therapy. There are also some alternative or additional treatments like yoga, massage or acupuncture.

However, timely and early diagnosis of symptoms of asbestos-related diseases is imperative for the effectiveness of the treatments.

5. Is Asbestos Dust Exposure Harmful?

When the materials that contain asbestos are disintegrated or damaged during its mining or processing, or when the buildings containing asbestos in their constriction materials are demolished or renovated, they release asbestos fibers into the air. These fibers contain asbestos dust. Hence, this asbestos dust consists of 2.26% to 63.8% of asbestos.

When this dust containing fibbers are inhaled, they easily get stuck in the throat, then windpipe and eventually the airways in the lungs and chest. They start irritating the cells in the lungs eventually causing symptoms like shortness of breath, extremely painful coughing, blue coloration of the skin because of lack of oxygen, and clenching of the chest.

This can lead to deadly diseases like lung cancer, mesothelioma, throat cancer, gall bladder cancer, brain tumor, ovary cancer, etc. It can also lead to some noncancerous disorders like asbestosis, pleural disorders, autoimmune disorders, etc.

6. What is Considered a Brief Exposure to Asbestos?

Brief exposure of asbestos would mean being exposed to asbestos at very low levels or for shorter durations or maybe with low intensities. That would mean inhaling the asbestos fibers found in fewer percentages in air, water, and soil or inhaling the same randomly or irregularly at low intensities. Hence, the chances of occurrence of deadly diseases like cancers associated with the same also become low.

However, along with the brief exposure if you are also a smoker or already have a weak immunity or health condition, then that requires early and precautionary diagnosis of the consequent diseases that may happen later. This is because these disease symptoms show up much later when the disease is in its advanced stages.

It can take many years to find out whether brief exposure was harmful enough or not. It can basically have a cumulative effect on the person later in life.

7. What is the Cancer from Asbestos Exposure?

According to the U.S. Department of Health and Human Services and the International Agency for Research on Cancer, Asbestos has been proved to cause cancer. This is because, with each exposure of fiber, the cell mutates within the body which if not treated timely can evolve into cancer. It can majorly cause lung cancer and mesothelioma.

Lung cancer is a disease in which the lungs get inflamed that causes painful cough, difficulty in breathing, clenching of the chest, blue coloration of the skin due to lack of oxygen and eventually lung damage.

Mesothelioma can be gastrointestinal or colorectal cancer or even throat cancer, kidney cancer, esophagus cancer, and gall bladder cancer.

These cancers are caused when large quantities of asbestos fibers are either inhaled or ingested by the person. These are majorly based on the occupation of the person. Some occupations lead to high levels of exposures of asbestos leading to higher chances of cancer development.

8.   Cancer from Asbestos Appears After How Long After Exposure?

After Asbestos exposure, the cancer is usually diagnosed after a very long period of time from the time of the exposure. It usually ranges from 10 to 50 years. The time duration depends on the following factors: -

- The duration of asbestos exposure whether its short term or long term.
- The intensity of the asbestos exposure whether it's low level or high level.
- The gender of the patient male or female.
- The type of cancer- lung cancer or Mesothelioma or throat cancer, gallbladder cancer or ovary cancer or brain tumor.

Because of this long-range of time, by the time people are diagnosed with this disease, they are aged between 60 yrs to 70 yrs.

Symptoms like difficulty in breathing, pain in chest and fatigue do not show up until the disease is in advanced stages. However, it is advisable to go for clinical tests at least 5 years after the exposure for the early diagnosis of the same in case the person was in an asbestos-exposed occupation.

9.   What is Known as Blue Asbestos Exposure?

Crocidolite asbestos exposure is also known as "blue" asbestos exposure. This is an almost opaque mineral. It mainly comes from the mines. Most of the mining areas are found in Bolivia, South Africa, and Australia. Its fibers are known to be the thinnest, hence can be inhaled easily and can dwell even more conveniently in the membrane of the lungs than any other kinds of asbestos.

Once they are inside the body, these fibers become unbreakable thereby creating worse conditions for the lungs and abdomen that can be fatal. Some of the diseases that can be caused are asbestosis, lung cancer or mesothelioma.

Materials that contain blue asbestos were last manufactured in the 1960s in the UK. As the exposure to the same has been proved to cause the worse kind of cancer, mesothelioma, it has been removed from the old constructions and not been used currently.

10. What are the Early Signs of Asbestos Exposure?

The signs and symptoms of asbestos exposure vary from person to person depending upon the duration of asbestos exposure whether it's short term or long term, the intensity of the asbestos exposure whether its low level or high levels, the gender of the patient – male or female and the type of exposure. However, some of the common and early signs of the same are as follows:

- Swelling of the neck or face area or any other kind of unusual swelling.
- Difficulty in swallowing food.
- The rise in blood pressure.
- Traces of blood in sputum.
- A breaking sound while breathing – a physician usually hears the same by placing his stethoscope on the chest of the patient.
- Difficulty in breathing especially it gets worse after physical activity.
- Hypertension or stress.
- Abnormality in fingers.
- Loss of weight - considerable and unintentional weight loss.
- Loss of appetite.

11. What are the Dangers of Asbestos Exposure?

Asbestos exposure can cause serious health hazards. They can start from breathing problems or digestion problems and can even eventually lead to death if left undiagnosed or untreated. The severe diseases caused by the same are Lung Cancer and Mesotheliomas – In this, the fibers of the asbestos settle in the membranes of the lungs or abdomen thereby causing inflammation and eventually cancer. This can be caused by inhaling or ingesting the fibers.

Some noncancerous diseases can also be caused like pleural abnormalities, laryngitis, weak immunity, retroperitoneal fibrosis which eventually leads to kidney failure. It can also lead to the enlargement of the heart because of the restricted flow of blood through the lungs.

Some more cancers can also evolve if cancer spreads from these parts to other parts of the body and not diagnosed or treated properly like throat cancer, gall bladder cancer, ovary cancer, brain tumor, etc.

12. The Exposure to Asbestos Dust Can Cause What Cancer?

Exposure to asbestos dust can cause lung cancer or mesothelioma. When the asbestos fibers are inhaled, the first stick to the throat, then windpipe, then the breathing tubes of the lungs. This may be cleared on its own if the patient coughs it up or swallows it. But in most cases, it goes to the endings of the tiny airways in the lungs and gets absorbed into the outer membrane of the lung or pleura. Pleura is the chest wall.

So on breathing, these fibers can cause irritation in the cells of the lungs or pleura. This consistent process eventually causes inflammation leading to lung cancer or mesothelioma.

If cancer spreads it can also lead to throat cancer, kidney cancer. The chances, stage, and type of cancer depend upon the type of asbestos exposure, the duration of asbestos exposure, age and gender of the person and smoking or non-smoking habits of the person.

PART 2

13. What are the effects of getting exposed to Asbestos dust?

When one is exposed to Asbestos dust, it becomes easy to get infected with Asbestosis. At the initial stage of exposure, it is very hard to suspect Asbestosis because the symptoms are mild and look like common medical conditions, which is why this is very dangerous. After a long period of being exposed to asbestos dust, shortness of breath and several forms of lung and tissue problems start showing up.

Certain types of cancers can develop in the body when one is exposed to asbestos dust. Mesothelioma is one of such cancers frequently associated with this, and it grows fast in the body due to asbestosis. Usually, it is the lungs that are directly affected, as they get scared and swell after with time.

Skin problems can also come as a result of being exposed to this dust. If the skin, at the time of making contact with asbestos dust, was not protected, it is almost inevitable for rashes, warts, and other complications to appear on the skin after some time.

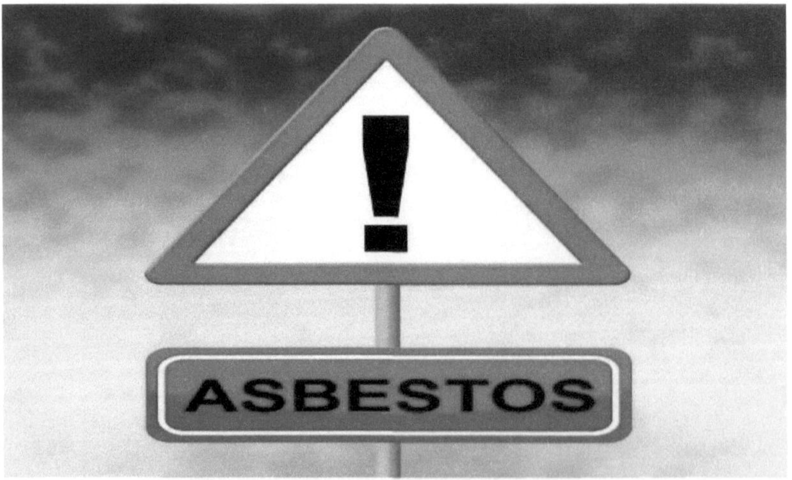

14. Is it possible to be infected by asbestosis symptoms?

Yes. Being exposed to asbestos dust is just as harmful to health as being exposed to the symptoms associated with the effects. If a person who has been exposed to asbestos dust comes down with an infection, it is best to not make contact until they are cured of the disease.

The different types of cancers caused by this dust are characterized by symptoms that make it easy for the disease to spread to someone who has not even been directly exposed to the dust. For example, if a person who works at a construction site starts to cough incessantly, all those around that person could be infected as well, since asbestos dust is usually present at construction sites and could be the reason the worker is sick.

15. Do small amounts of asbestos dust cause cancer?

There is actually no safe amount of asbestos dust exposure, even a little dust inhaled into the body can be very risky. This is because once asbestos dust is in the body, the inhaled particles find their way into the lungs and can get trapped there, which can result in serious health problems as time goes on.

The particles of asbestos dust are microscopic in size, so even if one tries to cough it out or swallow, there will always be some which did not make their way out of the chest cavity, this means that even the tiniest amount of dust can cause a lot of damage, including various forms of cancer. It is best to simply avoid inhaling asbestos dust no matter how small, it is far too dangerous no matter the amount.

16. Is smoking related to Mesothelioma?

Yes. Mesothelioma and other forms of cancer are related to smoking. It has been repeated time and again by health professionals that smoking is dangerous to the health and can make already harmful conditions worse. In the case of mesothelioma, smoking can make the condition deadlier and harder to cure. Researchers have said that a healthy person who is constantly exposed to asbestos dust and also smokes, has a 50 to 80 percent chance of developing mesothelioma, as well as other forms of cancer.

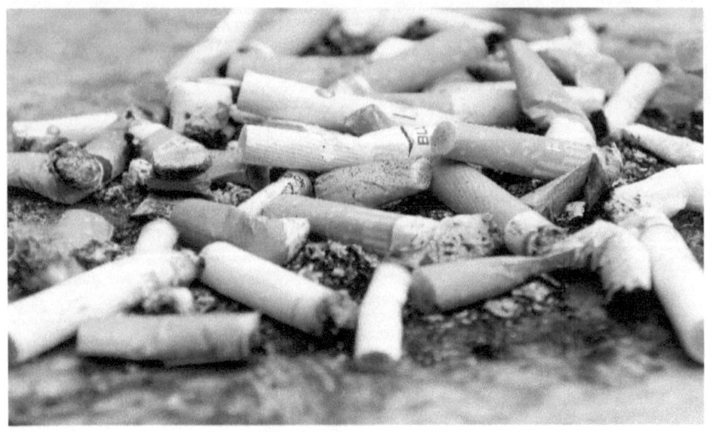

Asbestos dust directly affects the lungs, and a person who smokes already causes damages to the lungs, so when such a person is exposed to this dust, it is much easier for cancer to grow inside his or her body since the lungs are already getting weak due to smoking. This explanation can be seen in real life, as statistics show that mesothelioma and other lung cancers are more frequent in smokers than people who don't smoke.

17. What are the sources of Asbestos exposure?

There are many places where asbestos exposure can occur, this is because of how useful the compound is for the home and several work activities. Asbestos is resistant to fire and a lot of chemicals, so the manufacturing industry uses it a lot. This means that those who work in manufacturing industries or factories have a high chance of getting exposed to asbestos dust.

Construction sites also use asbestos a lot, so construction workers are exposed to the dust particles of this deadly compound. The automotive industry is not left out, they also use asbestos and the people who work there are at risk. All these industries show that one's place of work can be a source of asbestos exposure. Some products like tiles used in the home and office are made from asbestos products, so when they break, the dust is exposed into the air.

18. What are the symptoms of asbestos exposure?

When a person has been exposed to asbestos dust, certain symptoms are bound to manifest, some are immediate while others are long term. Initially, the dust particles get trapped in the throat and cause coughing and voice changes. When the dust is in a person's system, the chest cavity will receive it and the lungs will lose the ability to expand properly, this is what causes shortness of breath. There is also high blood pressure, noisy breathing, poor appetite, etc.

The skin can also become discolored due to a lack of proper oxygen circulation around the body. As the condition gets worse, the coughing will be accompanied by drops of blood and there will be constant chest pains.

19. What are the symptoms of Asbestosis and Mesothelioma?

After exposure to asbestos dust, the symptoms stated above will become more pronounced as asbestosis and mesothelioma start developing in the body. The most significant symptom is the shortness of breath felt by the patient. There is also a loss of appetite, which eventually leads to loss of weight. As the voice changes, there will be more intense coughing with drops of blood and headaches.

With mesothelioma, swelling is involved, that is why patients have swelling in the stomach, face or neck. The bowels also get blocked and skin tends to lose its original color as it starts getting blue. The fever, pain, coughing of blood and sputum are symptoms that look like other health issues such as tuberculosis, so it is best to approach a Doctor and not self-medicate if you experience any of these symptoms. The Doctor will recommend MRI scans and several tests that will show the real problems.

20. What diseases are caused by asbestos exposure?

The diseases caused by asbestos exposure are numerous, they are cancerous ones and non-cancerous ones, all of which pose a great danger to a person's health and life in general. The most common disease caused by asbestos exposure is cancer of the lungs, this is because the dust particles are moving from the nose or mouth straight into the lungs to cause damages.

Pleural disorders are also commonly linked to asbestos exposure. The pleura covers the chest cavity and lungs, which makes it a direct target of asbestos exposure effects. Mesothelioma is also a common disease caused by asbestos exposure, it is a type of cancer which affects the tissue of the abdomen and lungs. So far, this is the only disease known solely to be caused by asbestos exposure. There are also cases of lung scarring and other types of cancers associated with asbestos exposure.

PART 3

21. Is minimal asbestos exposure also dangerous?

Even small amounts of asbestos dust can be harmful to a person's health, so minimal exposure should be treated as if it is a lot of exposure. It is true that there is more danger to those who work in manufacturing, factories, automobile, and construction sites because they are exposed to the dust every day for a long period of time, but it doesn't mean those exposed to it for a short period of time are safe, the risks are just higher for those who inhale it for longer periods.

22. What is Multicystic Mesothelioma?

This is a form of mesothelioma, it is rare and almost always benign. The people affected by multicystic mesothelioma are women of productive age, and it can become malignant in extremely rare cases. Studies are still ongoing concerning the connection between asbestos dust exposure and this disease which occurs as clusters of cysts. It is not yet clear how exposure to asbestos dust leads to multicystic mesothelioma, but it is known to develop in the human body due to the introduction of foreign dust particles.

It usually occurs in women because their sex hormones trigger the growth of multicystic mesothelioma, and though chemotherapy treatment is a good method of curing it, the best solution is surgical because, with chemotherapy, the cysts are prone to regrow.

23. Will prolonged exposure to asbestos dust cause death?

When it comes to asbestos dust, prolonged exposure means that someone has been inhaling the dust for many years. If a person works at a place where he or she is constantly exposed to asbestos, there is a high chance of prolonged exposure, and also the problems that come with it.

There are many diseases, including deadly types of cancers which can kill a person, even if treatment commenced on time. So yes, prolonged exposure to asbestos dust can lead to the death of a person, more than a hundred thousand deaths have already been traced to prolonged occupations asbestos exposure. Apart from places of work, exposure can happen at any other place, like the home or surroundings that have materials made up of asbestos.

24. What risks are associated with asbestos exposure?

Asbestos exposure can be described as when a person swallows or inhales asbestos particles from any source. It is very harmful to health and can lead to severe sicknesses which could take a person's life. Since the mouth and nose are the main channels through which asbestos dust can enter a person's body system, the organs directly linked are the parts of the body most affected, so they are more at risk.

The nose directly takes the harmful dust particles into the chest cavity and lungs, so a lot of problems like lung cancer and mesothelioma can be the end result. The stomach, digestive, and metabolic systems are also at major risks because the toxic particles can find their way to that region through the mouth, that is why swelling of the abdomen, kidney issues, and skin problems affect a person who has been exposed to asbestos particles.

25. What is Asbestos exposure?

Asbestos exposure can be defined as the direct or indirect connection a person has with the dust particles produced by asbestos compound. The source of this dangerous exposure is usually where people work, so those who use asbestos materials in their production sites stand a high risk of inhaling this dust for a long period of time.

With reference to the source of asbestos exposure, it can be classified as primary or secondary. If someone is exposed to asbestos dust through the direct use of asbestos materials, then the exposure is primary. If a person who does not use asbestos materials gets exposed to the dust particles, it is most likely due to contact with another person who has been directly exposed to the dust, this is secondary exposure. A wife can get exposed to asbestos dust if the husband is a construction worker who uses asbestos materials.

26. Is asbestos exposure deadly?

Yes, asbestos exposure is deadly no matter the amount or duration of exposure, so it should be avoided by any means necessary. When studying how dangerous asbestos exposure is, there are two major factors to consider.

These two factors are; first, the amount of asbestos dust inhaled into the system. Secondly, the duration of time a person has been inhaling the deadly dust. Though no amount is safe to consume, an extended period of time spent inhaling the dust poses more danger to the human body. Also, even if the duration of time of exposure is short, certain factors can lead a person to inhale so much asbestos dust in a short while, this is very deadly and has immediate symptoms like coughing and tightness of the chest.

By default, people who smoke have a higher risk of falling sick and even dying a result of being exposed to asbestos dust.

27. How is exposure to asbestos dust treated?

When a person starts showing symptoms of asbestos dust exposure, it is best to see a doctor as soon as possible, and treatment has to start immediately after diagnosis. Due to the nature of the sickness caused by asbestos exposure, the healing process takes time and a lot of close medication.

The degree of the sickness due to asbestos exposure depends on a lot of factors, including a person's age, the source of that exposure, eating and drinking habits, if they smoke, etc. Medications like antibiotics, inhalers, surgery, therapy, and a lot more are used to treat the condition.

28. What is the relationship between asbestos and lung cancer?

Asbestos dust affects the respiratory system, so it is connected to the lungs directly. When dust is inhaled, it first gets trapped in a person's throat and causes immediate symptoms like change in the voice, chocking, and coughing. After which they move to the lungs and attach themselves to the tissues therein, causing scarring, shortness of breath, swelling, and a lot of other symptoms which are characteristics of lung cancer.

Usually, people who have been exposed to asbestos dust are expected to cough out blood and sputum when their lungs have been infected. This is also a symptom of tuberculosis and if a proper diagnosis is not carried out, a person with lung cancer might be getting treatment for tuberculosis, which is a lung disease with symptoms similar to that of lung cancer.

The lungs of a smoker do not function at an optimum level, so smokers are more susceptible to lung cancer when exposed to asbestos dust, even for a short period of time.

PART 4

29. How does asbestos affect health?

No matter the age, gender or medical history, a person who is exposed to asbestos dust is at risk of serious health problems that require long medical procedures for treatment. For women, ovarian cancer is a common effect of asbestos dust exposure as well as mesothelioma, but these cancers show up after years of exposure to the dust particles.

The immune system of a person can be seriously affected by the inhalation of asbestos dust, weakening the ability to fight infections, which is what gives way for all these diseases to take over the body. Inflammations, lung cancer, kidney failures, pleural effects, heart problems, and so much more can be the result of asbestos dust exposure.

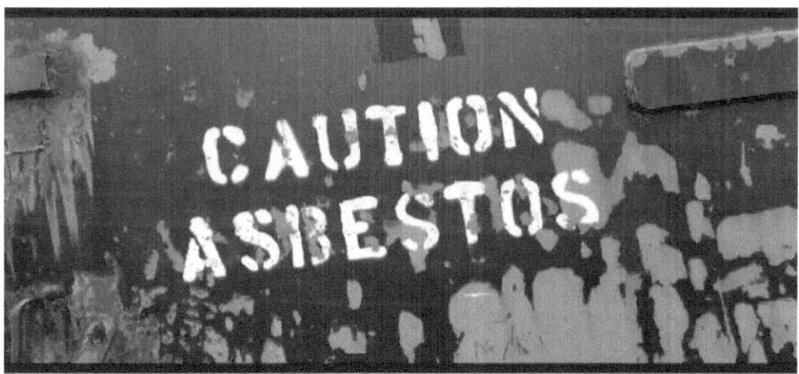

30. How fast can asbestos dust affect someone?

All things being equal, it takes time for someone who is constantly exposed to asbestos dust to feel the effects of the danger it has on their health. Even if the dust is inhaled in large quantities, the symptoms exhibited will be minimal and misinterpreted to mean regular cough or a result of fatigue. It can take up to 25 to 50 years of constant asbestos dust exposure before inflammations and malignant growths can start showing up, this is why treatment is difficult and time-consuming because the illness took a lot of time to develop into something fatal.

Due to the different lifestyles of each person, it may take shorter periods of time like 5 to 10 years for the symptoms to show up. For example, a smoker will definitely get infected faster and more severely than a nonsmoker. Also, those who go for regular random medical checkups can have their issues detected via blood tests and scans even if major symptoms have not started showing yet.

31. How long does it take for one to get Asbestos poisoning?

At first contact with asbestos, no poisoning can be detected, unless the dust was inhaled in very high quantity. Even at that, only coughing and other expected symptoms of ordinary dust inhalation will e exhibited, the real danger of asbestos dust takes time to grow on a person.

For those working at construction, factories, automobile, manufacturing, and regular blue-collar jobs, the chance of getting constant exposure to asbestos dust is really high. When the exposure has lasted for a period of five years, certain symptoms of asbestos poisoning can start to occur, as time goes on, the symptoms become more frequent and less treatable by regular painkillers or cough medications, this is when most people start going to the hospital for professional diagnosis. Our bodies differ, so the number of years it will take the poison to develop differs, lung cancer can take any time from 15, 25, 30, or even 50 years to grow in the body.

32. What are the symptoms of asbestos cancer?

There are many types of cancer that could result from asbestos cancer, some of which are cancer of the lungs, cancer of the ovaries, cancer of the gall bladder, cancer of the throat, cancer of the colon, mesothelioma which usually affects women due to their sexual hormones, and a lot more.

The sign of these cancers are shortness of breath, painful breathing, loss of weight and appetite, general body weakness, change in the voice, incessant coughing associated with sputum and/or blood, chest pains, chest tightness, noisy breathing, bowel obstructions, swelling in the abdomen associated with pain, constant discomfort, heartburn, ulcers, blood in the urine and vaginal discharge, and bloating. These are all signs that a person who has been exposed to asbestos dust might be infected with asbestos cancer.

33. How can you tell if your home is in danger of asbestos exposure?

Asbestos exposure is not only limited to places of work or office, but the home is also a source of exposure and this is how to know if you and your family are in danger; practice routine maintenance checks on your household products. Most of the materials that make up the house have asbestos as part of their constituents, so it is important to monitor such items and know when they are getting worse.

Your floor tiles, electrical outlets, pipes, roof painting, carpets, household insulations, and many other related materials are most likely made out of asbestos, so when they crack, the dust will be introduced into the air, endangering the entire family. So practice constant routine checks and quickly replace any material that is getting worse.

34. How do you know when asbestos is in the lungs?

There are no signs that asbestos has reached the lungs when someone is initially exposed to the dust, but as time goes on it can be seen in certain signs like inability to breathe and cracking sound in the chest when breathing. When an individual begins to see these signs, it means that the asbestos dust has reached the lungs and cancer or any other health disorder is already in the body.

35. What are the symptoms of Asbestos in the lungs?

When asbestos reaches the lungs, it causes many respiratory disorders like cancer of the lungs, mesothelioma, and other cancerous and non-cancerous ailments. These ailments usually show symptoms like continuous coughing associated with pain and headaches that last longer than three to four weeks, chest pains and tightness, coughing out blood or sputum, no desire to eat even when hungry, loss of weight, dryness of the throat and hoarseness of the voice, fever, etc.

All these symptoms mean that the lungs have been housing asbestos dust for a long time, and when the patient must get medical help as soon as possible.

36. What are the symptoms of Asbestos inhalation?

The dangers of inhaling asbestos can be deadly, that is why those who work in places where they are likely to inhale such dust should try to avoid it at all costs. When asbestos dust particles are inhaled, the symptoms experienced are coughing, chocking, the release of mucus, change in the voice and dryness of the mouth. This is because the throat is the first place the dust goes to settle before entering the lungs to cause more damage.

37. What are the symptoms of asbestos-related diseases?

A person can be suffering from a number of medical conditions, even if they are exposed to asbestos dust particles, this is why you should know the symptoms of asbestos-related diseases. The sure symptoms that prove a person who is exposed to asbestos dust is about to fall sick with lung cancer, ovarian cancer, abdominal issues, mesothelioma, colon cancer, skin problems, and other related conditions are constant coughing, snoring when there has been no previous record of such, abdominal pains and swellings, coloration of the skin to blue, painful urination which might be associated with drops of blood, shoulder pains, fluid in the lungs, chest tightness, inability of blood to form clots and obstruction in bowel movements.

38. What are the symptoms of Asbestosis?

Asbestosis is a condition whereby the lungs get scarred by ample deposits of asbestos dust particles which have been compiling in the lungs and chest cavity for a long time, usually over a period of five years. Asbestosis is not a cancerous disease but is dangerous. If it is not detected on time and left untreated or mistreated, it can lead to cancer of the lungs.

The symptoms of asbestosis start showing anywhere between 5 to 20 years of constant exposure to asbestos dust, they include blue skin coloration, chest tightness, cracking sound when breathing, stiffing of the lung tissues, etc. When these symptoms are detected, it is best for the patient to stop working because continued physical activity has been known to make these symptoms worse.

39. When was asbestos banned?

Asbestos has many beneficial uses in manufacturing and construction, that is why these industries always use it in their factories, but over the years, it has put workers in danger of occupational exposure to asbestos dust, making them susceptible to various deadly diseases, so the government had to intervene and ban the material.

The first major government intervention to the danger of asbestos started in the 1980s when the mining and production of asbestos were banned due to the failing health and death of workers. But over time, the banning of asbestos production did not look sufficient, so the ban was extended to the importation, sales, distribution, and even production of any materials that involved the use of asbestos.

Iceland was the first country to make this move, followed by more than 50 other countries in the world. Later on, the UK also banned asbestos in 1999, then in 2003 and 2005, Australia and all the counties of the European Union joined in banning asbestos and any material produced from it. This movement involved the removal of asbestos from places of work, offices, homes, and anywhere they could endanger people, but regular people were not advised to move them. Only licensed workers with the right training and personal protective equipment were allowed to move asbestos from places of danger to keep people safe.

40. Does asbestos cancer have a cure?

No. There is no cure for asbestos cancer yet, but that does not mean a patient will die. With so much advancement in science and technology, there is hope that in the near future, the cure for asbestos cancer will be discovered.

Despite being a permanent condition, there are treatment methods employed to help asbestos cancer patients with their symptoms. These produce lessen the severity of the symptoms and therapies help to slow down the growth of the cancer cells as well as prolong the life of the patient. There are antibiotics, aspirin, and other drugs which aid in helping asbestos cancer patients to feel less pain, inhalers are also prescribed to patients to allow them breathe normally without crisis at any time.

Surgical processes are also employed in managing asbestos cancer in different patients, for more advanced cases, chemotherapy and radiotherapy are also involved after surgery. The method a Doctor chooses to use for the management of asbestos cancer largely depends on the stage the patient was brought in for treatment, the earlier the case is brought to the attention of medical professionals, the greater the chances of survival.

PART 5

41. Is There an Asbestos Cancer Risk?

Yes, of course, there is certainly a possibility of a risk of cancer if a person is exposed to asbestos. Asbestos fibers when contacted through air or water or soil can lead to cancers like lung cancer, mesothelioma, ovarian cancers, throat cancers, kidney cancers, etc.

Basically, when each asbestos fiber contacts the cells of the body when they enter our body through the infected with asbestos air we inhale, the water we drink or the food we eat, the cells begin to mutate. This mutation eventually leads to cancers of various natures.

The type, stage and the likelihood of cancer depend upon the level and duration of exposure to asbestos. If the exposure has been for a very long time, the more the chances of developing cancer or if the occupation of a person has been such in which he is more exposed to asbestos-containing materials like construction materials, mining, shipbuilding, etc., then also the chances of cancer are higher.

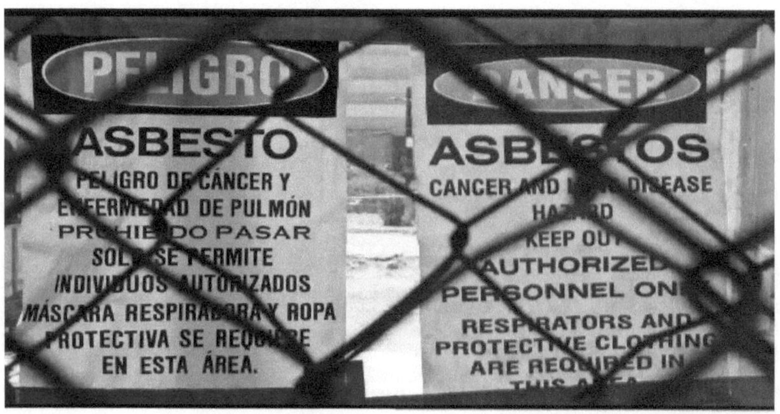

42. What are the Asbestos Caused Diseases?

The Asbestos caused diseases are listed below:

- **Mesothelioma:** This cancer is caused in the membranes of the following parts of the body: - Lungs — pleural Mesothelioma, Abdomen - peritoneal mesothelioma, heart - pericardial mesothelioma and Testicles. - Testicular mesothelioma.

- **Lung Cancer:** This is the most fatal disease. It is more common amongst people who are exposed to more quantities of asbestos for a longer period of time.

- **Asbestosis:** It is a noncancerous yet serious disease of the lungs. In this, the lung tissue gets scarred and inflamed. It restricts the lungs from fully expanding and relaxing itself leading to difficulty in breathing and clenching the feeling of the chest.

- **Pleural Effusions:** This is basically the fluids that are built up in the pleural region. It's a recurring but noncancerous disease that leads to severe pain and can affect normal breathing.

43. What Cancer Does Asbestos Cause?

Asbestos mainly causes occupational cancer. This is cancer caused to those people whose occupation is such that they are bound to get exposed to the asbestos environment or products containing asbestos.

The more a person is exposed to these occupations for longer durations or in larger quantities, the more are the chances of developing this cancer. Such occupations are like shipbuilding, mining, construction jobs, etc., the various kinds of such cancers are listed below:

1. Mesothelioma: It is one of the most severe kinds of cancers. This cancer develops in the protective membranes of the lungs, abdomen, heart or testicles.

2. Lung Cancer: It's also the most fatal and common cancer amongst asbestos-exposed occupations. Smokers are more prone to develop this cancer.

3. Ovarian Cancer: Women working in asbestos-exposed occupations are more prone to develop ovarian cancer. This cancer can develop when the asbestos fibers reach the ovaries through blood or lymph nodes or the reproductive organs.

44. What Causes Asbestos in a House?

Asbestos is a mineral that is used in the construction of buildings even houses because of some of its beneficial properties like insulation, malleability, etc.

This was majorly used prior to the 1980s in the US. It's not as harmful as such when it's a component of our house construction materials. But yes, it's dangerous when the house-made with asbestos-containing material gets damaged or is renovated.

This is because these processes lead to the release of asbestos fibers or asbestos dust particles when the materials are disintegrated, the air as follows:

- The damaging of the house through naturally occurring intense weather like strong winds, heavy rains or storms. This process releases dry and powdered asbestos within the house.
- The repair or renovation of the house includes tasks that break the asbestos materials like cutting the materials or scraping the wall plasters etc. This generates the asbestos dust particles into the air within the house.

45. What Causes Asbestos in Homes?

The construction materials of the homes do contain asbestos because of the various advantageous properties of this naturally occurring mineral. It is best used for insulators and is soft and malleable. This material is not harmful in its normal and good state.

However, if such materials are tampered with because of the processes like repair, renovation, remodeling or damage of the home, then that can cause the release of asbestos in the air of the home. This asbestos is released either in the form of fibers or even finer dust particles in the house which remains in the house for weeks after it is released as it is microscopic in size.

Because it's toxic in nature, it causes various deadly airborne diseases. Terraces, garages, and basements are the main areas in the homes likely to get exposed to asbestos. This could be because of old storage or water seepage in these areas. Also working on one's individual's vehicles in one's home garage itself can also lead to inhaling or swallowing of the asbestos fibers.

46. What is the Definition of Asbestos?

Asbestos in its natural state is a rock-forming silicate mineral. It's fibrous in nature. It consists of millions of thin fibers that can be released or disintegrated from asbestos on its scraping or damage. They are found in 4 colors – blue asbestos, white asbestos, brown asbestos, and green asbestos. Its advantageous physical properties are that it's soft, malleable, cheap and resistant to heat and electricity. It has been mined for almost 4000 years.

It was extensively used in building materials especially that required heat and electrical insulation. However, in the 20th century, its use has been restricted because of the various health hazards – cancerous and non-cancerous diseases - that it leads to.

The higher the exposure to the levels of asbestos in terms of its intensity and duration, the more are the chances of developing these diseases. The asbestos fibers or dust particles released in the air on its disintegration when inhaled or swallowed lead to these diseases.

47. What is Asbestos Poisoning?

Asbestos Poisoning means the health hazards caused by the human body due to its exposure to asbestos. When asbestos-containing materials are disintegrated or scarped or damaged, they become crumbled or powdered, thus, the thin toxic fibers or dust particles of the same are released into the air which when inhaled or unintentionally ingested lead to various kinds of cancerous and non-cancerous diseases.

These fibers are microscopic and can't be seen through the naked eye, so the individual will not realize or notice that he or she has actually swallowed or inhaled them.

Once they have entered the body, they would gradually start dwelling in the tissues, slowly developing into diseases like a slow poison whose symptoms also develop over a period of time usually appearing after years of contact with the asbestos. The 3 major diseases caused by those poisoned by asbestos are Mesothelioma, lung cancer, and asbestosis.

48. What is the Cause of Asbestosis?

Asbestosis is majorly an occupational disease that is caused to those who are in such occupations like mining of asbestos minerals, shipbuilding or other construction jobs which comprise of asbestos as one of the construction materials.

While in these occupations, when people are exposed to the asbestos toxic fibers or dust particles for a longer period of time and to the huge quantities of asbestos are more prone to developing asbestosis disease.

When the asbestos-containing materials break or disintegrate on its scraping, wear and tear or damage whether natural or manmade, they release microscopic toxic fibers and dust into the air which when inhaled, begins to dwell in the tissues of the lungs, thereby causing asbestosis. Though it's a noncancerous disease yet it's very dangerous. It basically leads to scarring and inflammation of the lungs leading to symptoms like difficulty in breathing, continuous cough, tiredness, pain in the chest, etc.

49. Which Asbestos Type is Dangerous?

The "friable" type of Asbestos is most dangerous. This is basically when the material containing asbestos mineral is scraped, damaged or disintegrated, it crumbled to a powdered form. This form can easily be released into the air and without our realization, we can inhale the same as its microscopic in size hence invisible to the naked eye. Such type of asbestos is found in ceilings, floor tiles, cabinet top shelves, fireproof doors, and other equipment, etc.

Whenever these are damaged naturally or manually they start releasing asbestos toxic fibers in the air in its friable form.

This is most dangerous as when inhaled, it first gets stuck in the mucus of the throat or the nose, then they reach the breathing tubes and eventually reach the tiny airways at the end of the lungs. Here they can't be removed by coughing etc. Hence they begin to dwell, slowly causing and developing dangerous diseases like Mesothelioma, lung cancer, asbestosis, etc.

50. Which is the First Symptom of Asbestosis?

Asbestosis is a noncancerous yet dangerous and fatal disease that is caused when one is exposed to asbestos-containing materials for a longer duration of time or in huge quantities. It mainly affects those who are in occupations that involve the use of asbestos-containing products.

When these products are disintegrated, broken or scraped through natural damage or manual tampering, they release dust particles into the air which are toxic and microscopic. Hence when they enter the body through breathing, they first get stuck in the mucus of the nose or throat, then the breathing tubes and eventually they start to dwell in the lungs.

This leads to the generation of the symptoms of deadly disease asbestosis. The first of its symptoms is Difficulty in breathing. This can perpetuate after physical activity but when the symptom persists it can happen irrespectively. It usually occurs unexpectedly or suddenly. This is a feeling where you feel suffocated as if there's not enough air to breathe. One is usually required to see a doctor immediately at the onset of this symptom.

References

Haspod. (2018, April 10). *When And Why Asbestos Was Banned In Uk Construction*. Retrieved from Haspod: www.haspod.com/blog/asbestos/when-why-asbestos-banned-uk-construction

Karen, S. (2019, August 30). *Cystic Mesothelioma*. Retrieved from Asbestos.com: www.asbestos.com/mesothelioma/cystic/

Karen, S. (2019, August 23). *Mesothelioma Death and Mortality Rate*. Retrieved from Asbestos.com: www.asbestos.com/mesothelioma/death-rate/

Matt, M. (2019, February 01). Retrieved from Asbestos.com: www.asbestos.com/occupations/auto-mechanic/

OSHA. (2019, May 14). *United States Department of Labor*. Retrieved from osha.gov: www.osha.gov/laws-regs/regulations/standardnumber/1910/1910.1001

The Department of Health. (2013, March 06). *When And Where Asbestos Used?* Retrieved from The Department Of Health: www1.health.gov.au/internet/publications/publishing.nsf/Content/asbestos-toc~asbestos-when-and-where

Tim, P. (2016, August 10). *Mesothelioma Cases Rise in Iceland Despite Asbestos Ban*. Retrieved from Asbestos.com: www.asbestos.com/news/2016/08/10/mesothelioma-cases-rise-iceland-despite-asbestos-ban/

Tonya, N. (2019, July 10). *Mesothelioma*. Retrieved from Mesotheliomadiagnosis.com: www.mesotheliomadiagnosis.com/asbestos/occupational-exposure

WHO. (2018, February 15). *Asbestos: Elimination of Asbestos-related Diseases*. Retrieved from who.int: www.who.int/news-room/fact-sheets/detail/asbestos-elimination-of-asbestos-related-diseases

WHO.(2019). *World Health Organization*. Retrieved from who.int: www.who.int/ipcs/assessment/public_health/asbestos/en